91888

Rheumatoid
Arthritis

D1246286

Rheumatoid Arthritis

◆

Everything You
Need to Know

Robert G. Lahita, M.D., Ph.D.

AVERY
a member of Penguin Putnam Inc. / New York

Most Avery books are available at special quantity discounts for bulk purchase for sales promotions, premiums, fund-raising, and educational needs. Special books or book excerpts also can be created to fit specific needs. For details, write Putnam Special Markets, 375 Hudson Street, New York, NY 10014.

a member of
Penguin Putnam Inc.
375 Hudson Street
New York, NY 10014
www.penguinputnam.com

Library of Congress Cataloging-in-Publication Data

Lahita, Robert G. (Robert George), date.
Rheumatoid arthritis : everything you need to know / Robert G. Lahita.
p. cm.
ISBN 1-58333-101-8
1. Rheumatoid arthritis—Popular works. I. Title.
RC933.L243 2001 2001022139
616.7′227—dc21

Printed in the United States of America

1 3 5 7 9 10 8 6 4 2

BOOK DESIGN BY JENNIFER ANN DADDIO

Contents

Introduction

"Rheumatoid arthritis? But I'm so young. How can I have arthritis?"

This is a common reaction when a patient is diagnosed with rheumatoid arthritis (RA). Many people think that arthritis of any form is a disease associated with aging.

But rheumatoid arthritis is not a disorder of aging or of wear and tear, as osteoarthritis is. In fact, RA is a common form of arthritis in children. The most likely cause of this disease appears to be a dysfunction of the immune system. It's not contagious and does not appear to be hereditary. In fact, it is not fully known just what causes RA. So what is this mysterious disorder? Who gets it? How is it treated? Will it ever go away?

This book was designed to answer the questions you may have about this disease and its impact on your life. It is based on the questions a countless number of my patients have asked of me, on questions I've heard at conventions and meetings, and on the overabundance of misinformation about the disorder that I read and hear daily.

This book was written strictly for people with RA. My goal was not to educate doctors (although many will find it helpful) but rather to address the very real questions that people with this disease have been unable to find. Unfortunately, the answers to many of the questions about RA are still unknown. But here you will find all of the information that is currently available on this disorder.

It is my hope that this book will provide you with the answers you seek and will aid you in your battle with RA. Read on as we attempt to solve the mystery of rheumatoid arthritis.

1

◆

Defining the
Disease

For many, a diagnosis of rheumatoid arthritis brings more answers than questions, as this is a puzzling disease that even the experts do not fully understand. In this chapter, I will try to explain to you just what rheumatoid arthritis is and the effects it has on your body.

What is rheumatoid arthritis?

Rheumatoid arthritis (RA) is a chronic inflammatory disorder of the movable joints. It differs from osteoarthritis in that it is not caused by wear and tear. Instead, it appears to be an autoimmune disorder—the body's own immune system produces antibodies against its tissues, causing inflammation and pain. Though it can be controlled, it can be progressive if left untreated. Most important, it is not a terminal illness if diagnosed early and treated appropriately. Generally, a disease such as rheumatoid arthritis affects people in the prime of their lives, striking most around the age of 40. A very important aspect of this disease is the way in which the joints are affected. It is a disorder of symmetry, which means that if your right wrist is affected, your left one will usually be affected as well.

Why is the disorder called rheumatoid arthritis?
Arthritis is inflammation of the joints. Rheumatoid refers to the muscles and bones.

What does "polyarticular" arthritis mean?
"Polyarticular" means that the arthritis affects many joints. As mentioned above, this disease affects many joints in a symmetrical fashion. Doctors often use this fact as a determinant for diagnosis. I will discuss this issue further in the diagnostic section.

Why is it considered to be a chronic illness?
This disease is called a chronic illness because it lasts for the life of the patient.

Just how common is rheumatoid arthritis?
This is one of the most common forms of arthritis. Its incidence varies among racial and ethnic groups, however. Approximately 1 in 100 Caucasians is diagnosed each year. It affects Asians at a much lower rate. Its incidence among the Japanese is roughly 2 to 4 out of every 10,000 people. Some groups of Native Americans, notably the Yakima, Pima, and Chippewa, have the highest prevalence rates at around 5 percent. Though the incidence of rheumatoid arthritis varies among races, its occurrence does not seem to correlate with where one lives.

Women are affected by rheumatoid arthritis three to four times more commonly than men. A major American study conducted in 1964 indicated that the prevalence was 3.8 percent among women and 1.3 percent among men.

Is it a relatively new disease?

Rheumatoid arthritis is one of the most common forms of arthritis. No one knows exactly when this affliction came into being, especially in North America. Since artifacts and skeletal remains indicate that the disease affected North American Indians several thousand years ago, the disease probably predated the arrival of the first explorers. Communicable diseases like syphilis may have been transported to this continent by European explorers, but that is not the case for rheumatoid arthritis.

Can rheumatoid arthritis be both acute and chronic?

In a sense, yes, it can be both. While ultimately it is a chronic disorder, its onset can occur suddenly, leading your doctor to believe that you have an infection in an affected joint. When a disorder flares up suddenly, rather than slowly progressing, its incidence is considered to be acute.

What are the symptoms of rheumatoid arthritis?

In rheumatoid arthritis, a joint becomes inflamed, which means it gets red and hot, sometimes filling with fluid and becoming very difficult to move. For the examining doctor, the signs of this inflammation would include warmth upon touching the area and swelling. On the other hand, the joint may be hot to the touch, but inflammation and redness may not be present. Inflammation, pain, and redness occur in all kinds of arthritic diseases.

When is a joint considered actively inflamed?

A joint is considered actively inflamed if it is tender. Swelling may be present around the joint or actually in the joint and is usually the result of fluid in the joint space.

What happens in the body to cause rheumatoid arthritis?

For reasons that are still unclear, the cells of the joints make inflammatory chemicals, and consequently fluid filled with even more destructive chemicals pours into the joint space. These chemicals promote the rapid and abnormal growth of tissue within the joint. This results in the destruction of bone along with cartilage.

What is genetics?

Genetics is the branch of medicine that deals with heredity, or the characteristics that we get from our parents and other ancestors. Certain characteristics, both favorable and unfavorable, are passed down from generation to generation through the code in our genes called deoxyribonucleic acid (DNA).

How is genetics important to RA?

As with all diseases, it is important to determine whether RA is inherited. This would allow doctors to predict which family members would likely get RA based on the present genes.

Is RA inherited?

Rheumatoid arthritis is not a classically inherited disease, so we cannot predict who will get the disease. There is, however, an association—although a slight one—between a certain set of genes found on chromosome number 6, or the immune response chromosome, and those who get this chronic disease.

What is HLA?

HLA stands for human lymphocyte antigens. These are molecules that are unique to each person and are found on the surface of one's cells. This is how the body distinguishes self from nonself. HLA is also called the major histocompatibility complex (MHC).

How is HLA important to rheumatoid arthritis?

Scientists have been looking for a genetic link to rheumatoid arthritis for years, and the obvious place to look was at the genes on the number 6 chromosome—the genes that control the immune response.

Why is RA more common in women?

One of the most perplexing aspects of RA is that it is about three to four times more common among women than among men. Most of the autoimmune diseases—and RA is the most common—are more prevalent in women.

What is a hormone?

A hormone is a chemical secreted from a gland in one part of the body that is transported via the bloodstream to affect the actions of cells, tissues, or organs in another part of the body.

Which hormones play a role in RA?

The female sex hormones, estrogens, appear to have the most effect on rheumatoid arthritis. They are thought to have a beneficial effect. Though estrogens are found in both sexes, there is more estrogen in women than in men. Estrogen stimulates immune cells.

Can birth control pills affect RA?

It was originally found that the incidence of RA was lower in patients taking estrogen-containing birth control pills, but they have not helped to improve RA symptoms as evidenced in careful research where women were specifically placed on birth control pills to prevent or alleviate RA symptoms.

Does pregnancy help to alleviate the symptoms of this disease?

Pregnancy helps to alleviate all the symptoms and signs of RA. In fact, this observation is nothing short of miraculous. I have seen women whose pains and aches disappeared with pregnancy. Some women have even told me that they would like to get pregnant for relief! I do not advise this, however.

What is the cause of RA?

No one knows for sure exactly what causes RA. Several possibilities have been contemplated over the years, including such infections as the Epstein-Barr virus, parvovirus, Lyme disease, and malaria. However, while these infections may produce symptoms similar to RA, none seems to be the actual cause.

What is Lyme disease?

Lyme disease is an arthritic illness that mimics RA and is caused by a spirochete (a corkscrew-shaped bacterium) called *Borrelia burgdorferi,* which is usually transmitted by deer ticks.

What is parvovirus?

Parvovirus is a type of DNA virus and is the cause of a childhood infection called "fifth disease" or the "slapped cheek" syndrome. In adults, this condition may cause joint pain that may last for weeks or even months. Though this condition's symptoms may mimic RA, parvovirus is not the same disorder nor does it cause RA.

What is the Epstein-Barr virus?

Epstein-Barr virus is the herpes virus that causes infectious mononucleosis. It has also been suspected as the cause of chronic fatigue, though there is little evidence to support this notion.

Is RA caused by any infection?

Scientists have considered infection as a possible cause; in fact, trials of treatment with the antibiotic tetracycline seemed to help alleviate the symptoms of rheumatoid arthritis in some patients. But there is far too little research in this area thus far, and results have been inconclusive. Scientists are also trying to determine if perhaps some type of bacteria may be the cause.

2

♦

Understanding the Immune System and Inflammation

Rheumatoid arthritis appears to be an autoimmune illness due to the presence of antibodies without evidence of infection. Autoimmune illnesses are those disorders in which the immune system, which is designed to protect the body from foreign invaders or germs, attacks its own body. In this chapter, we will explore just how the immune system works and what goes wrong and thereby causes the inflammation of rheumatoid arthritis.

What is the immune system?

The immune system is the component of the body—including blood cells, organs such as the spleen, and glands—that is designed to protect the body from harmful influences that are present within and outside of it. The immune system is extremely sophisticated; we are only now beginning to fully understand the various aspects of immune function and to realize that the more we uncover concerning function, the more complex the system is.

What are the components of the immune system?

The immune system is made up primarily of three categories of cells—the B lymphocytes (commonly called the B cells), the T lymphocytes (commonly called the T cells), and the phagocytes. These three groups of cells are the soldiers of the immune system, designed to protect the body from foreign invaders, commonly called antigens.

What is an antigen?

An antigen is any substance, including germs, bacteria, viruses, and fungi, that the immune system recognizes as foreign. In other words, an antigen is any substance that can trigger an immune response—an effort made by the immune system to rid the body of unwanted foreign invaders. An antigen can even be something that is part of the body that the immune system fails to recognize as self. In rheumatoid arthritis, the immune system does just that: It produces antibodies to cells or tissues that make up your body. It can make antibody to just about anything—even other antibodies. When the immune system makes antibodies against its own body, it is called an autoimmune response. In the case of rheumatoid arthritis, the antigen is another antibody. The resulting antigen-antibody combination is commonly called a rheumatoid factor. It remains unclear why these self proteins are seen as antigens in those suffering from rheumatoid arthritis.

What is an antibody?

An antibody is a protein made by cells of the immune system in response to a perceived foreign invader. Antibodies are produced by the B cells in response to the presence of antigens and bind to the antigen, carrying it to the spleen, where it is destroyed and eliminated from the body.

What are autoantibodies?

Autoantibodies are those antibodies made against healthy tissues of the body—presumably to eliminate them. There are only a few autoantibodies seen in rheumatoid arthritis as compared with other autoimmune diseases. This actually helps the doctor make the diagnosis.

What are immune complexes?

When antibodies attach themselves to antigens, the resulting union is called an immune complex. This complex is eaten by scavenger cells called phagocytes. These cells usually ingest the immune complex. When ingested by a cell, an immune complex is treated like a foreign substance and goes directly to the spleen to be eliminated. The spleen is the site where the foreign substances are taken apart and some of the antibodies are recycled.

What are lymphocytes?

Lymphocytes are a type of white blood cell. They are the main cells of the immune system. There are different categories of lymphocytes, such as T cells, B cells, and natural killer cells. All of the cells have a purpose, such as attacking and swallowing foreign materials, making antibodies, or killing other cells infected with virus particles. These cells have amazing capabilities, and new functions for them are discovered every year.

What are T cells?

T cell stands for thymus-derived lymphocyte. There are several varieties of T cells. Some (called the helper T cells) help immune function by telling the B cells to begin producing antibodies to fight off antigens. Suppressor T cells turn off immune function. Killer T cells (also called cytotoxic T cells) directly recognize, attack, and destroy antigens.

What are B cells?

B cells are very specialized lymphocytes that are responsible for a variety of functions. Their major role is that they eventually develop into cells called plasma cells, which make antibodies. The B cells got their names from a gland in chickens, called the bursa of Fabricius, where they were first discovered.

How does the immune system produce antibodies?

While the immune system produces antibodies as a response to antigens, it begins their production shortly before birth. While the antibodies of the fetus are limited in both type and number, there is evidence that they are produced in large amounts.

If a person is exposed to an antigen that is not recognized as self, his or her immune system rejects it as foreign. This process of recognition goes on every second during a person's life. When an individual becomes infected with any organism, an immune response results. After the immune response is made, a permanent memory is created in the immune system. One of the more fascinating things about the immune system is its ability to remember. As far as we currently know, there's only one other component of the body that can remember things—the brain.

The B cells are responsible for making the antibodies. They can be stimulated to make these proteins either directly by a foreign substance or by the T cells. When the B cells make an antibody in direct response to an antigen, it is called a T-independent response. When the T cells stimulate the B cells to make more antibodies, it is called a T-dependent response.

What is the relationship between B and T lymphocytes?

This relationship is one of the most important ones of the immune system. The T cells remember previously identified antigens and usually activate themselves and the B cells in the presence of antigens. Antigens are usually recognized by what are called antigen-presenting cells, also known as APCs. These cells are strategically placed in various parts of the body, such as the lungs, the liver, and the prostate. The APCs present the information, derived from a very complex process of recognition, to the T cells, which never forget an antigen.

In a more complicated series of steps, antigens can be presented directly to B cells. When T cells are activated, the B cells respond by specializing their efforts toward the foreign substance. They produce antibodies that target the specific antigens presented to them. This process is called differentiation.

What are phagocytes?

Phagocytes are white blood cells that eat other cells and certain waste products. The word *phagocyte* is derived from the Greek word *phagos,* which means "to eat." They are also called accessory cells.

What are macrophages?

Macrophages are large, mature phagocytes. These cells are essential to the function of the immune system. In some respects, they are also called accessory cells because they indirectly interact with the T and B cells of the immune system. Macrophages have many functions: They ingest and destroy foreign bacteria, diseased cells, and other cellular debris. They also send signals to lymphocytes to alert them to the fact that antigens are present. Macrophages are major producers of cytokines, the communication chemicals of the immune system.

What are leukocytes?

Leukocytes are white blood cells. When antigens invade tissues, leukocytes often secrete various chemicals in an attempt to kill the foreign organisms. These chemicals cause inflammation in the area where they are secreted. The leukocytes are major players in rheumatoid arthritis because they cause much of the inflammation involved in the disorder.

Why is rheumatoid arthritis called an inflammatory disease?

The pain, redness, and swelling present in rheumatoid arthritis is a result of inflammation.

How does inflammation occur?

Inflammation is a result of a series of chemical reactions. When the immune system detects an antigen, the white cells trigger the release of inflammatory mediators—chemicals including prostaglandins, nitrous oxide, oxygen radicals, among others—to fight the antigen. These mediators cause pain, redness, and swelling in the affected joint.

What causes the inflammation in rheumatoid arthritis?

In rheumatoid arthritis, there is no obvious foreign tissue that triggers the inflammation. It is generally believed that this disease is not a result of changes in temperature or pressure or of microorganisms (at least that have yet been identified). There are countless theories of possible causes of RA. The presence of macrophages indicates that there is injury or invasion within the joint and gives the signal for inflammation to occur. Again, the problem in rheumatoid arthritis is that there is no known invader. For this reason, it is believed that it is an autoimmune disorder—the immune system sees the tissues of the body's own joints as an antigen.

What is pus?

Pus is a collection of dead white cells that have played a role in both the secretion of cytokines and the overall destructive process at the site of inflammation. In rheumatoid arthritis, pus rarely is seen because there are not that many white cells called to a joint. When pus is seen in any aspect of rheumatoid arthritis, it usually means that there has been infection.

Why is there redness and pain with inflammation?

Inflammatory mediators irritate, raise the temperature of, and cause blood to flood the affected tissue. This causes pain. The increased blood and fluid cause redness and swelling of the affected area. The whole point of inflammation is to make the environment uncomfortable for the invading organisms. The process maximizes the influx of cells and substances that will kill the foreign invaders.

What are prostaglandins?

Prostaglandins are hormonelike fatty acids that regulate many processes in the body and play an important role in inflammation. Blockage of these chemicals can put a real damper on the process of inflammation, and, thus, they are currently the target of the largest group of new drugs available. Blockage of this molecule is a multibillion-dollar business because it plays such an essential role in inflammation. Scientists have been trying for years to develop selective prostaglandin blockers that would block only those prostaglandins involved in inflammation and not those that regulate other bodily functions.

Where do prostaglandins come from?

Arachidonic acid is a fatty acid that exists in the membranes of cells. Enzymes called cyclooxygenase (COX) convert arachidonic acid into prostaglandins.

What is an enzyme?

Enzymes are proteins produced by the body that catalyze chemical reactions without themselves being changed. They are critical to all of the body processes from immune function to inflammation. They work like a lock and key. Each enzyme works on only one chemical: The enzyme is the key, and the receptor that it fits in—the compound on which the enzyme works—is the lock. The key is specific and fits only one lock. This lock-and-key phenomenon is relevant to most of the new therapies that are available for patients with rheumatoid arthritis.

How are these enzymes important in the cause and treatment of inflammation in rheumatoid arthritis?

Blockage of these little molecules is the basis for the actions of aspirin and the other drugs referred to as nonsteroidal anti-inflammatory agents (NSAIDs). The problem with the blocking of all cyclooxygenases is that there are untoward side effects. When you block all of them, you block both the bad (those involved in inflammation) and the good COXs at the same time. In the early 1990s, it was discovered that there was more than one COX. Currently there are two known COX enzymes. Scientists are wondering if there are more yet to be discovered.

COX-1 is involved in housekeeping functions. Inhibition of this enzyme results in such problems as ulcers of the stomach, bleeding, and loss of kidney function. COX-2 is present only in the inflamed tissue. Selective blockage of this enzyme results in the reduction of joint pain and redness. Moreover, it seems that the receptors for this enzyme can be blocked. Most of the new "wonder drugs" for arthritis are based on this enzyme and its receptors.

3

◆

The Musculoskeletal System

The joints allow you motion and flexibility. They are not just hinged bones that move at will, but rather lubricated, highly developed mechanisms that account for mobility and dexterity. Connected to the brain via nerves, muscles, and tendons, they are truly responsible for the activities of daily living. They are also prime targets of rheumatic diseases like rheumatoid arthritis.

What is the musculoskeletal system?

The musculoskeletal system is the structural support of the body. It is composed of your bones and the muscles, tendons, ligaments, and cartilage attached to the skeleton. The skeleton protects the organs of the body. The nerves and the muscles that attach to the joints are important to movement of the body, including lifting, running, and standing still.

The Joints

What is a joint?

A joint is the point at which two or more bones connect. These bones allow movement of the extremities. Fibrous tissues, cartilage, tendons, ligaments, and muscles connect them. Some, such as the elbows, knees, and those in the fingers and toes, move; others, such as those present in the skull, are immobile.

Are there different kinds of joints?

There are many different kinds of joints. For example, the joints between the plates of the skull are called synarthrodial joints. By adulthood, these joints are connected by a series of fibrous bands and do not move. Some joints are connected by cartilage and move only very slightly. Such joints are those of the vertebrae and in the front of the pubis of the pelvis. This kind of joint is called an amphiarthrodial joint. Probably the most important type of joints, at least for the purposes of a discussion about rheumatoid arthritis, are the diarthrodial joints. These joints are lined with tissue made up of synovial cells that produce fluid that bathes the joint. They are also called synovial joints and further can be classified as ball-and-socket, hinge, saddle, and plane joints.

All joints, except for those in the skull, can become inflamed at some point. Sometimes the space between the bones can fill with cells, fluid, and even germs. These problems are often the cause of, or the result of, arthritis.

What is the joint space?

The space between the bones is called a joint space. Fluid made by the cells lining the joint fills the joint space, or the joint can be filled with cartilage. When this fluid becomes inflammatory, the synovial cells assume an amorphous shape. This is called a "pannus." The pannus can actually eat away at the bone of the joint. It is like a benign tumor in many ways. In the arthritic diseases, the joint space is the site of most inflammation.

What is joint fluid?

Joint fluid is a lubricant for the cells lining the joint and bathes both them and the cartilage cells. This fluid is rich in nutrients and contains some very important lubricants, which stop friction in the joint space. Normal joint fluid is usually very clear and has a slight yellow tinge. The fluid will also "gel" upon standing and is rather thick or viscous.

What is the synovium?

A capsule surrounds the joint space. The inner lining of this capsule is called the synovium, or the synovial membrane. It is usually three cells thick and overlaps on itself.

What do synovial cells do?

The synovial cells act as the major chemical and structural support cells for the joint. They also make up a small immune system within the joint. Some of the cells that make up the synovial membrane can eat germs, some make enzymes within the joint, and some are involved in the synthesis of the synovial fluid that bathes the joint.

Why is the synovium important in RA?

As rheumatoid arthritis progressively worsens, the synovial cells increase in number, and the lining itself gets very thick. The germ-eating synovial cells, in particular, increase. Usually these cells make up about only 20 percent of the synovial cells, but when rheumatoid arthritis is present, these cells increase to encompass 50 to 80 percent of the total synovial cells. The resulting mass is called a pannus. There is also an influx of T cells and the B cells to the area, indicating that there is a severe infection or that there is "cellular confusion" and really no identifiable foreign substance. The latter theory is probably the case, since there seems to be an overwhelming response to an unknown insult that triggers this disease process.

Bones and Tendons

What is bone?

Bone is the hard connective tissue that composes the skeleton and holds us upright. The muscles, tendons, and nerves depend on the bone.

How does RA affect bone?

Rheumatoid arthritis causes erosion of bone. The bone that surrounds the joint is most affected by this process.

What is a tendon?

Tendons are a very strong type of connective tissue that attach the muscles to bone. They allow the muscle to pull the bone as it contracts.

Can RA affect tendons?
Yes, RA can have a terrible effect on tendons, causing them to weaken, get inflamed, and even break apart.

What is osteopenia?
Osteopenia is a reduction in bone mass. This is not to be confused with osteoporosis, which is a condition marked by the progressive decrease in bone mass. Osteopenia is generally recognized as the beginning of osteoporosis.

How does the doctor test for osteoporosis?
The doctor can do a bone density (also known as a DEXA—dual energy X-ray absorptiometry) scan to see if your bones are normal for your age. You can also get a blood test to measure by-products of bone growth, which can confirm a diagnosis of osteoporosis.

Are osteoporosis and osteopenia seen in RA?
Yes. In fact, one of the earliest signs of trouble in the RA patient's skeleton is what is called periarticular osteopenia, a condition in which the bone around the joint is often "bleached" of calcium, giving it an empty appearance. This is usually the result of severe inflammation. The chemicals of inflammation come in to the bone area and actually bleach the bone of mineral.

4

◆

The Effects
of the Disease

Rheumatoid arthritis affects the body in many ways. This disorder involves much more than simply arthritis. This chapter will describe all of the symptoms that patients with rheumatoid arthritis may experience.

Is RA a disease of "old people"?

No, rheumatoid arthritis is quite common in young men and women. The mean age of development of rheumatoid arthritis is somewhere around the age of 50.

Is this a lifelong disease?

Since the exact cause of rheumatoid arthritis is unknown, a cure is not yet possible. For this reason, it is a lifelong disease. RA is, however, a very treatable illness. In fact, an increasing number of new therapies are currently being developed for the treatment of this illness. It pays, therefore, to do everything in your power early on to stop the progression of the illness.

Might the joints in my neck be affected?

RA of the thoracic spine (chest) and the lumbar spine (the lower back) is very rare and is usually associated with another illness. However, the spine in the neck area can be greatly affected. Early on, the neck can get very stiff and even lose some range of motion.

What about my shoulders?

Loss of motion of the shoulders is a common finding in RA patients. In fact, the shoulders can become frozen in place. The pain is worse at night when you are sleeping because the movements during sleep stretch the tightened joint capsule. This capsule gets really tight when there is extra fluid in the shoulder joint, which is not always obvious to the doctor.

How are the elbows affected?

Inflammation in the elbows is easily detected. Because a number of nerves pass through the elbow, a variety of confusing symptoms develops, including weakness of the pinky finger and numbness of the fourth and fifth fingers. Moreover, as the disease worsens, the elbow can become immobile and stay in a flexed or bent position until properly treated.

What happens to my hands in RA?

In all patients with rheumatoid arthritis, the wrists are affected. In fact, if the wrists do not appear to be involved, I would not diagnose a person as having RA. The knuckles and the middle finger joints are usually involved on both hands. Some changes that may occur in the hands include what doctors call ulnar deviation, which is the bending of the fingers toward the outer part of the arm (where the ulnar bone is located). The so-called "swan-neck deformity" is very typical in hands affected by rheumatoid arthritis. Here, the middle joint of the finger bends down and the joint nearest the tip of the finger bends up, giving the finger the appearance of a swan's neck. This deformity is very typical of the rheumatoid hand. The hand can also have what are called "boutonniere deformities," in which the middle finger joint pops up, resembling a boutonniere.

Swelling of the various ligaments around the wrist can result in trapped nerve syndromes like carpal tunnel syndrome, where the median nerve that goes through a closed space into the wrist is compressed. Another syndrome, also the result of nerve entrapment, is ulnar-nerve compression syndrome at the elbow. This causes extreme weakness of the pinky finger.

Sometimes rheumatoid nodules form on the tendons of the hands and may rupture. Tenosynovitis, inflammation of the tendons and the linings of the joint and tendon spaces, can also affect the hands. This can result in a rupture of the tendons and loss of mobility of fingers or, in severe cases, of the entire hand.

What happens to my hips?

The hips can certainly be affected by RA but not early on. Initially, the only symptom affecting the hips might be an inability to put on socks, stockings, or shoes. Later in the disease, the hip can be very inflamed and severely affected.

How might the knees be affected?

The knee is often the site of inflammation and joint destruction in RA. In many cases, the patient cannot bear weight on the knee. Since the knee is such a big joint, it fills with fluid and becomes hot and even noisy when it is bent or flexed.

Treatment usually involves removing fluid from the knee in order to help make a diagnosis and later to make the patient comfortable.

What is a Baker's cyst, and how is it related to RA?

A Baker's cyst is a fluid-filled sac that can develop behind the knee in those with rheumatoid arthritis.

How might my feet and ankles be affected?

The foot is a real nest of problems when the patient has RA. These joints bear a lot of weight, which means that they are particularly prone to complications. Many patients say they feel like they are walking on marbles early in the morning. Many experience a burning sensation on the soles of the feet. It is also common for patients to have difficulty keeping their feet straight or to be unable to wear shoes because the toes flex upward. The knuckles where the toes join the foot are particularly prone to inflammation and deformity. Consequently, the gait of some RA patients is grossly affected.

Can I get nerve entrapment syndromes in my feet?

Yes, the foot also has various nerves and tendons that can be affected by swelling and inflammation. This "crunching" of nerves causes the common burning sensation on the bottom of the foot when you walk or stand in one place for a long time.

Disease Outside of the Joints

What other systems can be involved?

As with other autoimmune diseases, RA can affect almost every other system of the body. This includes the heart, lungs, kidneys, eyes, skin, nerves, blood, and gastrointestinal tract.

What does RA do to the eyes?

The eyes and the mouth can become very dry in patients with rheumatoid arthritis. This problem, which is actually the result of inflammation, is called sicca syndrome. The "white part" of the eye, or the sclera, is most affected by RA. Inflammation of this tissue is called episcleritis. This problem is usually relatively benign without causing many long-term problems; however, rarely, a formation similar to a rheumatoid nodule develops on the surface of the eye, which can perforate the eye and cause blindness.

How does RA affect the throat?

First, there can be inflammation of the joints of the neck. In addition to the neck pain, the voice can be affected, and occasionally pain can be felt on swallowing. Most of these problems are worse in the morning.

How might my lungs be affected?

Most of the lung problems in RA are not apparent to the patient and may only be picked up on a routine chest X-ray. Small round masses called pulmonary nodules can be found in the lungs of some patients. Inflammation of the lining of the lung also can occur and cause pain on breathing. Patients can be slightly short of breath, but because they limit most of their physical activities anyway, this is not very apparent. All of these symptoms usually respond to anti-inflammatory therapy and other treatment drugs.

Does RA affect the kidney?

The filtration mechanisms of the kidney are not affected in RA patients like they are in autoimmune diseases like lupus. In fact, most of the problems involving the kidneys in patients with RA are the result of the drugs taken for treatment of the disorder.

How can RA affect my heart?

The tissue encasing the heart, or the pericardium, can get inflamed, causing some pain and discomfort. Most patients do not notice this, however. When rheumatoid nodules affect the heart—as they can in rare instances—the electrical system of the heart, the functions of the heart valves, and the actual heart muscle itself can be affected.

Can RA affect my stomach?

Most of the complications involving the gastrointestinal tract are the result of drug therapy. The drugs used to treat arthritis can block the protective chemicals in the stomach and cause ulcers. Sometimes, however, the complication of dry mouth can be so bad that it can cause ulcers to form in the mouth.

What skin manifestations might I experience?

Vasculitis, or inflammation of small blood vessels, is a common problem affecting rheumatoid arthritis patients. Vasculitis can cause the appearance of "snakelike" vessels on the skin that are quite tender to the touch. Rarely, it can cause ulcers to form on the heels, around the ankles, and on a person's shin bones.

Can the drugs I take cause skin changes?

They most certainly can cause problems in the skin. Some of the drugs used to treat the condition can cause large bruises on the skin. Small hemorrhage spots called petechiae can also develop.

How are the nerves affected in RA?

The nervous system is very susceptible to problems because of RA. As mentioned above, entrapment syndromes are very common as a result of rheumatoid arthritis. In addition, vasculitis can develop in the covering of a nerve, causing a weakness or dysfunction of a limb or other part of the body that seems to be unrelated to other possible contributors, such as nerve compression or malpositioning of a limb. This can result in major problems if left untreated. In this particular case, the nerve might actually have to be biopsied.

What happens to the spinal cord in the neck in RA?

This is one of our biggest worries. When the cervical, or the neck, bones have arthritis and inflammation, there is the risk of the spine becoming unstable. A simple X-ray will confirm whether the spine is at risk for damage. Damage to the neck spine results in weakness of the extremities, or even paralysis. Destruction of the spine nerves bears no relation to the amount of pain felt by the patient, so damage can ensue without any warning. Suddenly, subtle signs and symptoms of damage, including weakness or loss of feeling in the arms or legs, just appears.

What is amyloidosis?

Amyloid is a form of protein with a small bit of sugar attached. This material deposits in organs and tissues in people with chronic disease, particularly rheumatoid arthritis, causing problems. It can infiltrate organs, resulting in dysfunction.

What does RA do to my blood?

Patients with RA have anemia, or low red-blood-cell count. This is not due to blood loss, but rather because the bone marrow, where red blood cells are produced, is affected by the disease, and thus the cells are not made efficiently. This is called anemia of chronic disease. There is no amount of vitamin or iron that will successfully raise the blood count to normal in a rheumatoid patient.

What is Felty's syndrome?

This is a serious and little understood disorder that can occur as a result of RA. Patients with severe nodule-forming RA generally get this syndrome. The white cell count drops, the spleen enlarges, and some patients get leg ulcers. Sometimes lymph nodes enlarge, and the patient's platelet count drops precipitously. Fortunately, aggressive therapy with disease-modifying anti-rheumatic drugs (DMARDs) often causes complete resolution of this symdrome.

Other Disorders That Can Be Confused with or Mimic Rheumatoid Arthritis

What are some of the other diseases that can mimic RA?

Any disease that causes the joints to become red and hot can be mistaken for RA. Some of these conditions include Lyme disease, bacterial blood infection in the joint, infection with parvovirus, German measles, sometimes AIDS, hepatitis B, rarely crystal formation in the joints as occurs with gout, and palindromic joint disease.

What is palindromic rheumatism?

Palindromic rheumatism is arthritis that occurs in cycles. The disease goes away completely between attacks. An episode can last a few hours or a few days. The disease is usually treated with a disease-modifying drug like sulfasalazine or gold. Other anti-inflammatory agents may be used as well.

Will my RA go into remission?

It certainly can go into remission over time after the diagnosis is made. Doctors look for specific criteria to determine if a patient's RA is in remission. At least five of the following criteria must be present before the doctor can say that the disease is in remission.

1. The duration of morning stiffness must be less than 15 minutes.
2. Absence of fatigue.
3. Absence of joint pain.
4. Absence of joint tenderness upon movement.
5. Absence of swelling in joints and tendons.
6. Sedimentation rate must be less than 30 in women and less than 20 in men.

How do I get into remission?

This can happen by itself or as a result of therapy.

What can I do to function better?

In short, you can begin to take the many anti-inflammatory agents or DMARDs that are on the market. Chapters 7 and 8 will tell you about all of the options available for treating your symptoms, including, drugs, surgery, physical therapy, and alternative therapies.

5

♦

Juvenile Rheumatoid Arthritis

One of the most difficult diseases to diagnose in children is juvenile rheumatoid arthritis (JRA), the most common cause of arthritis in children. This is because there are numerous childhood ailments that must first be discounted. This chapter will explain some of the peculiarities of JRA.

What are some of the symptoms of juvenile rheumatoid arthritis? How does it differ from the adult form of the disease?

The juvenile form of RA is quite different from the adult form. It can be very debilitating in children, causing fatigue, weakness, and severe pain in the joints. The clinical presentation can be anything from inability to play with other children to doing poorly in school. When suspicious of something, the pediatrician can get the appropriate X-rays or laboratory tests to make the diagnosis.

In children, the disease really becomes a collection of signs and symptoms of other diseases, some of them quite scary until the diagnosis is solid. For example, the child can present with pauciarticular arthritis (the most common form), which means very few joints are affected, as compared to the systemic form (the least common form), where many joints are involved, along with other systemic symptoms such as fever. The joints must be affected symmetrically—on both sides simultaneously—as is the case in adults. Finally, there is the polyarticular form of arthritis (occurring in about half of the children with the disease).

Erosions occur, and their manifestations are far more serious in children, since their bones are still in development. For example, the development of the jaw can be stunted due to inflammation, causing a small lower jaw, a condition called micrognathia. Often a limb's growth may remain stunted as the child grows older. One of the most serious complications of JRA is overall stunted growth.

What are the diagnostic criteria for JRA?

Juvenile RA is diagnosed in children 16 years of age and under. The child must have persistent joint pain with inflammation that makes movement very difficult for at least six weeks, and other forms of childhood arthritis first must be excluded.

Is it easy to misdiagnose a child with this disease?

Yes, it is very common to misdiagnose children with this illness. That is why physicians must follow strict guidelines in its diagnosis.

What is systemic JRA?

Systemic juvenile RA causes such symptoms as high fever of about 101°F or greater once or twice a day. These are called fever spikes. A pale pink rash that does not itch is commonly found on the chest. Boys and girls are affected equally, and the peak age of onset is usually between 1 and 6 years of age.

What are some of the clinical problems associated with systemic JRA?

Besides the rash and the fever, there is profound joint pain. The child's lymph nodes may be enlarged, and there may be inflammation over other areas, such as the lining of the lung or the heart. This can cause pain on breathing or lying down. There can be an increase of the white blood cell count or the platelets and a major rise in the sedimentation rate. To further confuse the doctor, the patient usually has no positive rheumatoid factor. The child's spleen and liver often enlarge. When the fever goes away, the arthritis resolves and the child can get better. In rare instances, there can be severe complications, but early treatment and diagnosis of this condition are critical.

What is polyarticular JRA?

Polyarticular juvenile rheumatoid arthritis is arthritis in five or more joints. About 40 percent of the children with JRA have this form and often have rheumatoid factor in their blood.

Peculiarly, this rheumatoid-factor-positive form of arthritis is found mostly in little girls around 8 years of age. Boys do get this form of JRA, but girls outnumber them three to one. These little girls often have bone erosions, many nodules, and a more aggressive disease than the children without the rheumatoid factor. In that regard, this form of JRA resembles the adult form more than any other. These children often experience fatigue, listlessness, growth retardation, blanched bones (osteopenia), loss of appetite, and often extreme and unexplained weight loss.

What is pauciarticular JRA?

In pauciarticular JRA, arthritis is present in four or fewer joints. This form is usually categorized as early onset or late onset. Early onset pauciarticular JRA strikes very young—usually around 1 to 5 years of age—and affects girls primarily at a ratio of four to one. The late onset form strikes children over the age of 5 and occurs mostly in boys. It is characterized by pain and inflammation of the large joints and the tendons and ligaments.

What eye problems affect those with JRA?

For some reason, children with JRA can experience severe irreversible eye changes that include everything from cataracts to partial visual loss. Eye problems occur most commonly in children with early onset pauciarticular disease, although they can affect any child with JRA. The eye problems begin with painful red eyes and occur in four out of five children with pauciarticular JRA. Children with JRA should have their eyes examined regularly.

Are autoimmune antibodies evident in these children?

Yes, for some reason the antibodies found in lupus and other autoimmune disease are found in these children. This does not mean that they have lupus, just that this syndrome is likely to be an autoimmune disorder, like adult RA. The occurrence of these antibodies in children with these diseases can sometimes cause scary confusion.

A good pediatric rheumatologist knows the importance of eliminating other illnesses as causes of symptoms.

What are the lifelong consequences in children?

Many patients require lifelong therapy with anti-arthritic drugs. The anti-inflammatory agents and the new disease-modifying anti-rheumatic drugs (DMARDs) are very useful in the later life treatment of JRA patients. Problems like stunted limbs or a shortened jaw are only a few side effects of JRA. Today, these skeletal deformities are not as prevalent since early diagnosis and treatment are much more common. Unlike many other aspects of the disease, these growth changes can be irreversible.

What type of doctor should my child with JRA see?

Specialists called pediatric rheumatologists would examine, diagnose, and treat your child. They are experts in the childhood forms of arthritis.

6

♦

Making the
Diagnosis

Making a diagnosis of rheumatoid arthritis is not easy. As with all other diseases, there are many ways that your disease might manifest itself. In addition, the first complaints might be very general and vague. The doctor initially tries to develop a differential diagnosis—one made by comparing and contrasting the symptoms of different disorders. Once the doctor suspects rheumatoid arthritis, he or she will look for the typical signs and symptoms of the disease. When enough of these signs are present, the doctor may order a few laboratory tests to confirm his or her diagnosis of RA.

Unfortunately, there is no one specific test for rheumatoid arthritis, but the presence of certain findings on more than one test can confirm a positive diagnosis. This chapter will explain some of the tests a patient may have to undergo.

The Clinical Evaluation

What are the clinical signs of rheumatoid arthritis?

There are many clinical signs of RA. Chief among them is what doctors call arthralgia or, "joint pain." As the disease progresses, the arthralgia worsens and eventually becomes arthritis, or inflammation of the joint, which makes movement very difficult. Morning stiffness exacerbates this problem.

Are there criteria for a diagnosis of RA?

Yes, there are seven criteria a doctor looks for when establishing a diagnosis of RA. At least four of the following seven criteria must be present in order to make the diagnosis. If any of the first four are present, they must have been present for at least six weeks.

1. Stiffness in the morning that usually lasts for longer than an hour and gradually improves over the course of the day.
2. Inflammation, pain, and swelling of three or more joints at the same time.
3. Pain and inflammation of the hand joints (wrist, knuckle, and/or those in the middle finger).
4. Arthritis on both sides of the body at the same time (symmetry). This does not have to be the case with arthritis in the hands, where some of the smaller joints might not be affected in both hands.
5. Nodules over the bony parts of the joints or next to them.
6. Presence of the antibody called rheumatoid factor in the blood.
7. Evidence of bone erosions or early bleaching of bone on X-ray.

What does symmetry mean?

This refers to the fact that the corresponding joints on each side of the body are affected. The presence of symmetry helps the diagnostician confirm a case of rheumatoid arthritis.

Describe the morning stiffness associated with RA.

Morning stiffness is a critical sign. The joints are very difficult to move upon arising in the morning and for at least an hour thereafter. As the day gets longer, the stiffness goes away, although it may not clear entirely. This symptom often helps the physician differentiate RA from other types of arthritis, since in osteoarthritis the patient generally gets stiffer as the day goes on.

How long might the stiffness last?

In the worst case, you can be stiff all day. Most patients complain of being stiff in the morning for over an hour. Stiffness degree and duration can vary among patients.

How many joints are usually affected by rheumatoid arthritis?

This is a very important question. Generally, when only one joint is swollen or painful, it is not RA. Isolated inflammation is usually the result of infection or a type of arthritis caused by crystal formations like gout, but not RA. There should be at least three or more joint areas involved to make the diagnosis of RA. These three areas should also have swelling (from fluid) and even perhaps be warm to the touch (from inflammation).

Which joints are important in RA?

In RA, the diarthrodial joints, or those that have a space between them and move, are the ones that are most affected—this means those joints like the jaw, the wrists, elbows, and those in the hands and feet. When a doctor examines a patient with the disease, he or she looks for symmetrical involvement of the joints of the wrist and the hands, though not every sore finger joint has to mirror one on the opposite hand. The knuckles of the hands and the toe joints are the most commonly affected.

Are the hands very important in RA?

Yes, arthritis of the hands and wrist helps make the diagnosis. A swollen wrist or swollen knuckles are very important factors when making the diagnosis of RA.

Is fatigue common in rheumatoid arthritis?

Fatigue is very common in the early and late stages of RA and may reflect the overall body inflammation present along with low-grade fever, aches, and pains that lead to numerous complications like depression and lack of sleep.

What is fibromyalgia?

Fibromyalgia is a condition characterized by generalized soft-tissue achy pain and stiffness. This condition is common in those with RA and is felt in addition to arthritic pain. It is often dismissed as being "all in one's head" because of the vagueness of the symptoms, but it is a very real, very painful condition.

How is fibromyalgia diagnosed?

The pain must be widespread—felt above and below the waist and often on the left and the right sides of the body. In addition, there must be pain in the spinal bones of the neck or back or in the chest. There also may be low back pain. The doctor looks for trigger points of pain—eighteen areas of the body where, when pressure is applied, pain is felt in those with fibromyalgia. Pain—not just tenderness—must be felt in at least eleven of the eighteen pressure points to confirm a diagnosis of fibromyalgia.

Do patients with RA feel pain every day?

Not after your doctor places you on therapy; however, before that—you bet! Your days and nights may be filled with pain resulting from the inflammation and bone destruction taking place in your body. "Get thee to a specialist!"

What is a rheumatoid nodule?

A rheumatoid nodule is a small, firm bump that usually appears on the tendons but can occur anywhere. They are the result of inflammation. Nodules are sometimes biopsied to make sure that they are only rheumatoid nodules, but they are rarely surgically removed. They are not malignant and rarely cause dysfunction. As a rule, they do not cause pain or infection.

Scientists generally call these nodules foreign-body reactions. They are akin to what would happen after a large splinter lodged itself in your skin. The only problem with RA is that no apparent foreign body is evident that would produce these nodules.

Not everyone with rheumatoid arthritis gets rheumatoid nodules, but when they are present they can help confirm a diagnosis of RA.

Who gets rheumatoid nodules?

About one-fifth of RA patients get rheumatoid nodules. Other people with diseases like lupus can get nodules, but this is rare.

Will they go away?

The rheumatoid nodules generally go away with treatment of the disease. In fact, they are great indicators of disease activity and good barometers of clinical response to treatment.

Is it important to start therapy early?

Absolutely! The sooner the diagnosis is made, the sooner that we can prevent the joints from getting progressively inflamed and becoming destroyed. Remember that the process of destruction in rheumatoid arthritis is quite significant. Patients have actual erosions of the bones in their hands, feet, and other joints. Consequently, the earlier the disease can be diagnosed, the earlier it can be treated.

Blood Tests

What role does the laboratory play in the diagnosis of RA?

The laboratory has a limited role in the diagnosis of RA. Unlike a disease like lupus, where patients make antibodies to several components of the body, the patient with RA has almost none. The only antibody that is common in patients with rheumatoid arthritis is the rheumatoid factor. Other antibodies may be present, but they do not necessarily indicate RA. In addition to the presence of antibodies, there are other laboratory findings that doctors may look for to help them diagnose RA, including anemia (low red blood cell count) and other blood cell count abnormalities. During the course of treatment, doctors often have to monitor the patient's health with laboratory tests, as several of the drugs used to treat RA can affect the health of many organs.

What is the rheumatoid factor?

The rheumatoid factor is an antibody directed against another antibody in the blood. It is present in about 60 percent of rheumatoid arthritis patients; however, its presence does not automatically indicate RA, as it is common to other disorders as well. Conversely, the absence of rheumatoid factor does not rule out a diagnosis of RA. When the rheumatoid factor is present in a RA patient, one is said to have sero-positive disease. When there is no rheumatoid factor, an RA patient is said to have sero-negative disease. Generally, sero-positive disease is more aggressive than sero-negative.

What is an ANA?

ANA stands for antinuclear antibody. This antibody is directed against the nuclei of certain cells.

Is an ANA present in those with RA?

Some RA patients have antinuclear antibodies, though the strength, or titer, of such antibodies is low. They are more common to other autoimmune conditions, though doctors must not overlook the possibility of rheumatoid arthritis when they detect ANAs. Too often doctors hastily make a diagnosis of lupus when they find ANAs without ruling out RA.

What is an ESR?

ESR stands for erythrocyte sedimentation rate. The speed at which red blood cells settle to the bottom of a test tube helps doctors check for inflammation. The faster these cells settle, the more inflammation is present. The ESR is the test conducted to determine the rate at which the red blood cells settle.

Imaging Studies

Are X-rays helpful in diagnosing RA?

X-rays are very useful in making the diagnosis of the various forms of arthritis. They can help confirm a doctor's suspicions of rheumatoid arthritis and can enable doctors to find bone deformities, extra growths, thinned bone, bleached bone, or actual erosions of bone. Bone erosions are the most important findings in RA, as they are the hallmarks of this disease-causing process. One of the first signs of RA in a young person with early disease might not be erosions but blanching of the bone around the joints. This condition is called osteopenia. When it occurs around the joints, it is called periarticular osteopenia. Doctors look for this early on. I usually get X-rays of the hands of patients that I suspect have RA, and I look for osteopenia and erosions.

Are there other imaging techniques that might help the doctor diagnose RA?

The plain X-ray film is really the best and least expensive way to diagnose RA. Other tests are good for ruling out specific problems that are of a greater magnitude and might require an extra look. However, the best imaging technique for RA is the basic X-ray.

What is an MRI?

MRI stands for magnetic resonance imaging. It is the use of a magnet to get the atoms in the area being observed to vibrate in order to produce signals, which are translated into images on the computer. MRI is useful for determining the density of tissues. This very complicated and somewhat expensive test should be reserved for special situations. It is most effective for looking at the "soft" tissues like the brain and the spinal cord. While it can be used to look at tendons, capsules of the joints, and bone, generally the plain X-ray film is just as effective and less expensive.

What is a CAT scan?

CAT stands for computerized axial tomography. CAT scans are an advanced type of X-ray involving the shooting of several X-rays from different planes and different vantage points around the area being viewed. The final image is viewed on a computer screen rather than on film.

What is a bone scan?

The bone scan is another technique for the imaging of bone problems. A radioactive substance is injected into the patient's arm. This substance sticks to bone and can be seen on an X-ray. Doctors can detect new bone growth based on the distribution of the radioactive substance on the X-ray. New bone can grow as a result of injury, infection, or inflammation. Bone scans are very useful in some patients where the diagnosis is not really solid. The most common radioactive material used in this process is technetium-99 (Tc99).

7

◆

Traditional Therapy: Drugs, Surgery, and Rehabilitation Therapy

While rheumatoid arthritis can be a devastating disease, you should not despair—there are several treatments available for this disorder. This chapter will introduce you to the medications and procedures used to treat RA.

Are there new and improved treatments available for RA patients?

Yes, there are many new agents for RA patients, probably more than for any other rheumatic disease.

Why are these drugs coming forth at this time?

Our understanding of RA is getting better each year. Before 1990, we knew very little about elements of immunity like the cytokines and the molecular mechanisms that affect the actual disease process. Only in the past few years have we become familiar with the chemical changes that occur in diseases like rheumatoid arthritis and lupus.

NSAIDs

What is an NSAID?

NSAIDs is an acronym for nonsteroidal anti-inflammatory drugs. As the name of this class of drugs indicates, they relieve pain by reducing inflammation without steroids. The NSAIDs block several enzymes that make the chemicals that cause inflammation.

Have they been around for a long time?

NSAIDs were first discovered in the 1960s. The first one was phenylbutazone, an agent no longer in use. (Aspirin was really the first NSAID, but some doctors and scientists do not classify aspirin as an NSAID, but rather as a salicylate.) NSAIDs had such remarkable effects on patients that they were copied and perfected until newer, less toxic agents were developed.

What is aspirin?

Aspirin, or acetylsalicylic acid, is one of the most remarkable drugs ever developed. It is among the oldest of medical pain relievers. While it is technically a nonsteroidal anti-inflammatory pain reliever, some do not classify it thus, but rather as a salicylate. For the most part, it accomplishes the same results that NSAIDs do but is much cheaper; however, so much aspirin is necessary to achieve the same results as the newer NSAIDs that the side effects are too much to handle for most patients.

Can NSAIDs be dangerous?

NSAIDs are quite dangerous when they are misused. In fact, the use of over-the-counter NSAIDs has resulted in quite a few deaths from misuse. NSAIDs are remarkable relievers of pain and inflammation, but they can also cause kidney failure, bleeding ulcers, and even meningitis. The development of newer agents began due to the fact that over 16,000 people died from NSAID use in 1997 in the United States alone.

So, is it safe to take these agents?

It is safe to take drugs if you are aware of the potential problems. Most of the time, patients have no problems with these drugs. If they do experience difficulties, they should inform their doctor who will prescribe a new drug or switch them to a safer drug like the COX-2-selective agents.

What are the most common side effects of the NSAIDs?

The most common side effects of NSAIDs affect the gastrointestinal (GI) tract. Patients may experience ulcers, bleeding, and perforations. One of the more common findings is simple upset stomach, or dyspepsia. Diarrhea is also common. Most of the side effects occur in the elderly or in other high-risk groups; however, I have seen healthy people who were unable to tolerate NSAIDs. Some of the other effects that have been observed include kidney failure, easy bruising and bleeding, and a rise in liver enzymes in the blood coupled with a loss of appetite. Some patients actually develop hepatitis and have to be hospitalized. In rare instances, patients can suffer liver failure.

Can the NSAIDs ruin my kidneys?

You bet. This is particularly true of people who have bad kidneys to begin with. The elderly, the dehydrated, and those taking drugs that cause dehydration are all at risk of encountering problems with these drugs. There is some evidence that the NSAIDs can lower the filtering capacity of the kidneys.

Are over-the-counter drugs different from those prescribed for me?

No, the over-the-counter drugs are the same as the prescription agents, just at lower doses. Several years ago, it was decided that certain NSAIDs could be offered over the counter at a lower concentration. Unfortunately, this did nothing to lower the potential for abuse (some people take these like candy) or lower the incidence of bad effects. Ibuprofen (Advil, Nuprin, and others) has the potential for causing problems like ulcers in the stomach, perforation of the bowel, and bleeding if the directions for its use are not followed.

What is a COX-2 drug?

This is a new class of NSAIDs. A COX-2 drug is one that selectively blocks cyclooxygenase-2 while leaving cyclooxygenase-1 alone. Before the discovery of COX-2 drugs, anti-inflammatories blocked both COX-1 and COX-2. While both of these enzymes play roles in inflammation, COX-1 also has several "housekeeping" roles in the body, including regulating normal cell function in the gastrointestinal tract and the blood. So blockage of this enzyme, while eliminating pain and inflammation, can cause harm to the intestinal wall over the long term. The mucous coating of the stomach is destroyed, and thus there is a great likelihood for the development of ulcers and major problems with gas and discomfort. You can even vomit blood or have black, tarry stools. It might be wise to look for these signs if you have to take large amounts of NSAIDs as a matter of course.

There are only two COX-2-selective drugs on the market: Celebrex (celecoxib) and Vioxx (rofecoxib).

I heard that more than two COX enzymes might exist. Is that true?

I would like to think so. In fact, I wonder if there is a COX-3 and a COX-4, with specific roles to play in other organs.

Are the new drugs more expensive?

The new COX-2 drugs are rather expensive—a 30-day supply of Celebrex is $84 and of Vioxx is $72. A 30-day supply of Motrin costs $22.50 and Naprosyn $52.20. Because these newer drugs are more expensive, your health maintenance organization is liable to deny you access to these safer agents. The worst factor is that Medicare patients—those who usually need it most—have no access to these very expensive safer drugs unless they pay for them out of their own pockets.

Is managed care a problem concerning availability of these agents?

This really depends on your insurance plan. Generally, if you can prove that you have had some problems tolerating the old class of nonselective COX agents, your insurance company should approve the COX-2-selective agents for you. Symptoms of intolerance include persistent upset stomach, evidence of ulcers, and nonrelief of pain or inflammation.

How do the COX drugs affect the bowels?

These drugs have both bad and good effects on the small and large intestines. COX inhibitors can cause diarrhea in some people; however, they can also reverse and destroy colon polyps and possibly prevent colon cancer itself. I would not be surprised if COX-2 inhibitors are prescribed for everyone in the future as a protective measure for bowel cancer, particularly if one has a relative with colon cancer.

So, these drugs can help me in cancer prevention?

Yes. These drugs do some remarkable things that have just become obvious to scientists. They accelerate a process called programmed cell death (apoptosis). This acceleration speeds the death of malignant or potentially malignant cells. Currently, these drugs are the subjects of research in cancer of the colon, stomach, and breasts.

Do these drugs cause high blood pressure?

All of the prostaglandin inhibitors, those agents that inhibit COX, can raise the blood pressure or in rare cases even lower it.

Can NSAIDs cause swelling in my legs?

The movement of substances like sodium, an essential mineral, through the body relies on good kidney function. Data show that the NSAIDs can cause sodium to be retained at least for a short time, since this may change with continued use of the drug. If sodium is retained, leg swelling as well as elevated blood pressure may ensue.

What effects can NSAIDs have on my brain?

Evidence from ongoing studies shows that NSAIDs, particularly the COX-2-selective agents, improve thinking and the overall condition of patients with Alzheimer's disease. Although research into this aspect of therapy with these drugs is still incomplete, it is clear that improvement in thinking does occur. This, by the way, has nothing to do with inflammation in the brain with this disease, since cortisone given to patients with Alzheimer's disease has no effect.

Are NSAIDs addictive?

While NSAIDs are very effective at relieving pain, they are not narcotics and are not addictive.

Can I use NSAIDs for the treatment of conditions other than arthritis?

Yes, these drugs are good for many other problems besides arthritis. For example, NSAIDs can be used to ease pain after surgery, to relieve the pain of sports injuries, and to effectively ease menstrual pain and headaches. Some doctors even use them to relieve pain in patients with cancer. These are just some of the uses of these new drugs.

Might I be allergic to NSAIDs?

Yes, some people are allergic to aspirin. These people may experience wheezing and shortness of breath and develop hives after taking the drug. The presence of nasal polyps can suggest allergy to these drugs.

What NSAIDs might be prescribed to me for the treatment of my rheumatoid arthritis?

There are numerous such NSAIDs. Here is a list of the most common. The generic name is listed first, followed by the common brand names in parentheses.

- aspirin, enteric-coated (Ecotrin)
- aspirin, extended release (Zorprin)
- celecoxib (Celebrex)
- choline magnesium trisalicylate (Trilisate)
- diclofenac (Arthrotec, Voltaren)
- diflunisal (Dolobid)
- etodolac (Lodine)
- fenoprofen (Nalfon)
- flurbiprofen (Ansaid)
- ibuprofen (Motrin)
- indomethacin (Indocin)
- ketoprofen (Orudis, Oruvail)
- meclofenamate sodium (Meclomen)
- meloxicam (Mobic)
- nabumetone (Relafen)
- naproxen (Naprosyn)
- naproxen sodium (Anaprox)
- oxaprozin (Daypro)
- piroxicam (Feldene)
- rofecoxib (Vioxx)

- salsalate (Disalcid, Mono-Gesic)
- sulindac (Clinoril)
- tolmetin (Tolectin)

DMARDs

What is a DMARD?

DMARDs stands for disease-modifying anti-rheumatic drugs. Most DMARDs take a long time to begin working. In addition, because these are such strong agents, you must be carefully monitored by your doctor while taking these drugs.

Name some DMARDS that can be helpful to me.

There are many DMARDs that are helpful in the treatment of rheumatoid arthritis, including Plaquenil (hydroxychloroquine), Rheumatrex (methotrexate), Imuran (azathioprine), Cytoxan (cyclophosphamide), Arava (leflunomide), and Azulfidine (sulfasalazine).

Aren't some of these drugs used in chemotherapy for treating cancer?

In some instances, these drugs are useful for the treatment of various cancers. They interfere with the division of cells and can be useful in treating tumors. In the treatment of arthritis, we are trying to accomplish the same thing—the obliteration of the cells responsible for the disease process.

What is hydroxychloroquine?

Hydroxychloroquine is a drug used to treat malaria. A brand name for this drug is Plaquenil.

Is hydroxychloroquine useful in treating RA?

It is moderately useful in the treatment of RA.

How does it work?

Exactly how it acts in the treatment of diseases like RA is not known. This drug is known to act as a mild suppressor of the immune response and gently even thins the blood in some studies.

What is the usual dose?

The standard dose of the drug is 200 milligrams twice a day. It becomes most effective about three to six weeks after you begin to take it.

Is it used in the treatment of other rheumatic diseases?

Hydroxychloroquine and a similar compound chloroquine are used for the treatment of diseases like lupus, Sjögren's syndrome, and antiphospholipid syndrome.

Is it safe?

It is considered one of the safest DMARDs available. Serious adverse effects are rare.

What are some of the side effects?

Occasionally, patients may experience visual problems including change in pigmentation of the retina of the eye or some loss of feeling of the cornea. An eye exam is recommended six months after starting the drug and every six months thereafter. Persistent nausea or an allergic reaction with itching and rash are also possible. All in all, this drug is quite safe and free of side effects.

What is methotrexate?

Methotrexate is a favored drug among rheumatologists for the treatment of RA. It interferes with a metabolic pathway called the folic acid pathway.

How does it work?

It interrupts the cycle of certain cells important to the immune system.

What is the usual dose?

Patients with RA usually begin with a low dose, usually 7.5 milligrams per week, followed by a gradual increase to 25 milligrams per week. Some patients can even tolerate higher doses. It is really up to your doctor. It should be taken with 1 to 4 milligrams of folic acid daily, as this vitamin limits the poisonous effects of the drug.

When does it start to work?

It usually takes effect within four to six weeks.

What side effects should I watch out for?

Some of the most common side effects of this drug include sores in the mouth, lung congestion, nausea, abdominal cramps, loss of appetite, and, although rarely, infections. Fortunately, these are not common, and most are reversible when caught early. In addition, new nodules similar to rheumatoid nodules form in some patients. Your doctor can treat these nodules with a drug called colchicine.

What is folic acid?

Folic acid is a vitamin that is usually supplemented in those taking methotrexate to reduce the side effects.

Who should not take this drug?

People with liver and kidney problems, diabetes, immune system disorders, and high alcohol intakes should not take this drug. Pregnant women, women intending to get pregnant, and nursing women should not be started on the drug. Women planning to conceive a child should wait at least one menstrual period after stopping methotrexate before trying. Men planning to father children should not take the drug both because it might affect fertility and because it could be harmful to the baby.

Does methotrexate interact with other drugs?

Yes, it does. Evidence exists that the new COX-2 drugs increase the blood levels of methotrexate. In fact, the elderly with decreased kidney function should not take the drug. Almost every NSAID will increase the potential for problems with this agent; however, under the care of your doctor, this should not be a problem. The doctor will test you periodically for potential problems.

What is sulfasalazine?

This is a sulfa-containing agent useful for the treatment of arthritis. It is not terribly toxic, but it has greater toxicity than hydroxychloroquine.

Can it be used to treat RA?

Yes, it is a good drug used in combination or by itself.

What is the dose?

The usual dose is 2 grams per day by mouth; however, your doctor will start you on a low dose to see how you fare on it. Some doctors will go to 3 grams per day, depending on any side effects experienced and how your arthritis progresses on the drug.

What are the side effects?

Rashes, loss of appetite, and nausea are side effects experienced with this agent. Serious reactions are rare and include hepatitis, a lupus-like disease, and even a decrease of sperm counts. Your doctor should watch for these. Men should notify their doctors if they plan on fathering children so that the drug can be stopped or replaced with something else.

What is Imuran?

Imuran (azathioprine) is an immunosuppressant that changes the DNA structure of certain cells.

Can it be used in the treatment of RA?
It is used for rheumatoid arthritis that is difficult to treat and does not respond to other agents.

What is the usual dose?
Imuran in a dosage of 1 to 2.5 milligrams is generally given per kilogram of body weight. If your doctor weighs you before beginning this agent, this is why.

What are the side effects?
Nausea, vomiting, belly pain, and occasionally hepatitis or problems with the making of blood cells are seen with this agent. If you also have gout and are taking the drug allopurinal (Zyloprim), make sure you tell your doctor, as your Imuran dosage will have to be adjusted.

What is leflunomide?
This drug's brand name is Arava. It is another drug that acts on the DNA of cells like the T cells. It is new and quite useful in the treatment of RA and is as effective as methotrexate or sulfasalazine.

What is the usual dose?
The doctor gives you a loading dose in order to get the blood levels of the drug up to therapeutic levels in your body: The patient is started with 100 milligrams per day for three days. After three days, the dose is lowered to 20 milligrams daily. If the patient tolerates the drug, the dose can be lowered to 10 milligrams per day.

What are the side effects?

Diarrhea is the most frequent side effect. Changes in the liver function tests, reversible hair loss, and a rash are all part of this drug's side effects.

Who shouldn't take this drug?

Women who expect to become pregnant and men expecting to father a child should discontinue the drug and replace it with cholestyramine for eleven days to bind up the drug and eliminate it. Your doctor can test your blood levels to make sure that it is out of your system before you get pregnant or father a child.

What is penicillamine?

Penicillamine (Cuprimine, Depen) is a chelating agent, which means that it binds metals in the blood and aids in their removal. It is very effective in treating RA, but it also has some toxicity, including muscle weakness, a lupus-like syndrome of the kidney (protein in the urine), and other effects on the blood counts. It is not related to the antibiotic penicillin.

Is it useful in treating RA?

This drug is modestly useful in patients with RA. It used to be the standard of care but has been replaced by newer agents.

How does it work?

It decreases the formation of antibodies, stops the white cells in their tracks, decreases the function of the T cells, and removes damaging molecules called free radicals.

Is gold used to treat RA?

Yes, gold therapy is an old remedy that still has a place in the treatment of RA. In fact, many doctors feel that gold therapy can induce a complete remission of the disease.

What are the forms of gold administered for the treatment of rheumatoid arthritis?

There are injectable forms of gold and an oral form. The oral form is less effective than the injectable form.

Are there dangers inherent in taking this drug?

As with all drugs, gold therapy has its problems. It may cause mouth ulcers, rashes, protein in the urine, and, rarely, low platelets (blood-clotting particles) and a low white cell count.

What is the usual dose of gold?

The usual dose of injectable gold is a test dose of 10 milligrams, followed one week later by 25 milligrams once a week for two weeks, and then 50 milligrams weekly for up to 20 weeks. It can be given longer if the patient has a dramatic remission.

Should I be watched on gold?

Your doctor will keep a record of your injections and test you before each new dose. The doctor will take urine and a blood count to make sure that all is well.

Can I take gold if I am pregnant or planning to conceive?
No.

Why should I take the injections if the oral dose is safer?
Although the oral dose may be safer, it is less effective. Moreover, there are more stomach and bowel side effects with the oral preparation.

What is Enbrel?
Enbrel is the brand name for etanercept, a modern biological response modifier.

How does it work?
There is a cytokine, or chemical messenger, present in the joints called tumor necrosis factor (TNF). This inflammatory mediator is one of the major problem-causing cytokines in RA. (It gets its name because it was found to cause weight loss and the shrinkage of tumors in young animals. Many years ago, it was actually thought of as a means of controlling cancer.) On cells there is a docking mechanism called a cytokine receptor. In order for cytokine (a chemical messenger) to do its job, it must join with a receptor. Enbrel is a laboratory-made receptor. Instead of docking at the regular receptor, the TNF sticks to the laboratory-made receptor Enbrel and is inactivated.

How do you take this drug?
Enbrel is taken by subcutaneous (under the skin) injection twice a week. Most patients administer the injection themselves. It is relatively easy once becoming accustomed to it.

What are some of the side effects?
There can be some local allergic reactions at the site of injection. You can also experience headaches, fever, low blood pressure, and upset stomach. If you develop an infection on the drug, you must call your doctor. You will probably have to stop the drug until the infection is treated and you are well enough to start it again.

How long do I have to be on it?
Until the disease is controlled. There are very few studies of long-term use, since the drug is fairly new.

How do I get it?
Your doctor should write a special prescription for you, and you will have to learn how to inject the drug from the doctor.

Is it expensive?
It costs anywhere from $8,000 to $12,000 per year. It is very expensive and out of range for many people. Your HMO will have to be coaxed into understanding why you need this medicine.

Can it be used with other agents?
Yes, it can be used with almost anything, including methotrexate.

What is Remicade?
Remicade (infliximab) also inhibits the actions of TNF, though it does it differently.

What does it do?

This drug is really an antibody against the TNF. It is made from both mouse and human protein. It is also called a monoclonal antibody because it is made from only one cell source.

How is it given?

Remicade is given intravenously by a doctor or a nurse.

Is there any danger to giving this agent?

The side effects are pretty similar to those experienced with Enbrel, but, in addition, your body can produce antibodies against the drug.

What do I do to prevent this from happening?

You usually have to take another immunosuppressant like methotrexate to prevent the development of new antibodies.

Is cortisone a drug used for RA?

Yes, cortisone is a steroid used for the treatment of rheumatoid arthritis, but it should be used sparingly, since patients may become dependent on it.

How did cortisone use for the treatment of RA come about?

One of the great physicians of the past, Dr. Philip Hench, noted that cortisone was a "cure" for RA back in the 1940s. In fact, it was so good that everyone with RA started to take the drug—until its side effects became apparent.

Does it really work?

Yes, cortisone will normalize the findings on X-rays. When the drug is stopped or decreased, however, there is the so-called rebound phenomenon, and the patient actually gets worse.

Are there times when this agent is indicated for RA?

Yes, this drug is given to treat the most severe forms of the disease, as when vasculitis or fluid around the heart with inflammation of the coverings of the heart is present. Occasionally, it is given to quell the severe pain and inflammation of a very hot joint. I occasionally give an intramuscular injection of cortisone to control an acute flare of RA. The key is to avoid long-term use of the drug.

What is cyclosporine?

Cyclosporine (brand names Neoral and Sandimmune) is an immunosuppressant that is very effective in the treatment of rheumatoid arthritis, but side effects like high blood pressure, drug interactions, and cost have limited its use.

When is cyclophosphamide used?

Cyclophosphamide is a very potent chemotherapeutic agent, which is used only for the most severe forms of rheumatoid arthritis. I have rarely used this agent to treat this condition. It has many bad side effects like hair loss, suppression of the production of bone marrow, and the later risk of cancer.

Don't all of the chemotherapy drugs have a risk of cancer later on?

Generally speaking, anything that suppresses the immune system has the risk of causing cancer. However, some agents that interfere with DNA synthesis run a higher risk of cancer development as the patient ages.

Can the above drugs be used in combination with each other?

These drugs are most effective when used in combination. Clearly somebody who does not respond to one drug like methotrexate by itself could respond to the addition of two other agents like sulfasalazine or even leflunomide. I find, for example, that people who fail to respond to methotrexate usually benefit from the addition of infliximab or etanercept.

What is plasmapheresis?

Plasmapheresis is the removal, cleansing, and replacement of the blood. In the case of rheumatoid arthritis, the removal of immune complexes and certain antibodies through plasmapharesis has resulted in some improvement of the patient's condition. This has not been impressive.

What is Adsorption for RA?

Columns that contain a substance called protein A absorb materials from the blood. In the case of RA, absorption of immune complexes and certain antibodies have resulted in marked improvement of the patient's condition. These treatments are very costly, and the number of treatments and long-term effectiveness of this kind of therapy is not known. This treatment also requires that you be in an office setting where it can be done or in a hospital. You would have to go to the hospital with some frequency to the short pheresis-stay unit.

Surgery

Is surgery a treatment option for RA?
Surgery can be very helpful in certain cases of RA. It is not for everybody, however, since any surgery involves risks. The doctor has to measure those risks in each case.

How are you considered for surgery?
A preoperative evaluation has to be completed by your doctor. The patient must be told the benefits of having surgery, and a good doctor will also let the patient know the downside of the surgery.

Is there anything that I should do before having surgery?
Yes, you should consider all the options and already have tried drug therapy, rehabilitation therapy, and modification of your daily activities to maximize your benefits.

If you have been on cortisone, you need to take a stress test before and during your operation. The adrenal glands of those people who have been on cortisone may not be able to cope with the stress of the surgery.

What are the biggest risks?
The RA patient presents a risk for nerve injury either before or during surgery, and this must be considered. Many RA patients are also at risk for infection in their joints either because of drug therapy or because of their poor state of health. The biggest risk occurs with patients with RA of the neck or, more specifically, at the base of the

skull. Such patients run the risk of total paralysis during surgery because of hyperextension of the neck during any procedure. The patient with this kind of disease has to be evaluated carefully, and the spine has to be made stable before the surgery.

How do I avoid this problem?

Ask your doctor. The doctor usually performs a complete neurological evaluation as well as extensive X-rays before surgery.

What are some other concerns?

If your doctor plans to replace or surgically correct many of your joints, he or she must plan the repair of the joints in order to maximize your ability to recuperate. A rheumatoid foot, for example, should be repaired before the knee to permit the foot to be used for rehabilitation on the knee.

What are some of the possible surgical procedures?

RA patients can benefit from teno-synovectomy, or the removal and reconstruction of the tendons and the linings of the joint. This is often performed on the hands and the feet. Today, joint replacement, removal of the synovium, fusion of certain joints, and surgical cleaning of the joint are all common surgical procedures performed on RA patients.

What is rehabilitation therapy?

Rehabilitation therapy is a way to maximize your daily functions. Chronic diseases, as well as surgery, can severely limit such function. You might not be able to do certain things like put on your shoes or your sweater or open doors. Rehabilitation therapy helps you maintain, preserve, and actually improve function of the affected joints by increasing the strength, endurance, and range of motion of the joint. It is also designed to teach you alternative methods of function. It is a means of getting back on your feet.

What is a functional limitation?

Functional limitation means simply that one's ability to conduct some day-to-day activities is impaired. It could apply to your job or your ability to perform activities at home.

Will I always be disabled?

No, not at all. Disabilities can be either temporary or permanent. If yours is permanent, you will just have to learn to use some other part of your body to compensate for the permanent problem.

What are the elements of a good rehabilitation program? What should I look for?

First, the goals should be realistic. The rehab specialist should carefully explain exactly what the plan of action is and what should be accomplished with this plan. Your program should be based on you and you alone. Everybody is different. Second, the period to achieve these goals of rehabilitation should be realistic. If it is going to take two years, you need to know that. Third, the rehabilitation specialist should consult with your arthritis specialist to make sure your program will not cause you further pain and deterioration. Fourth, you should be able to report your progress accurately and not overdo it. The doctor and you have to come to some agreement on your progress.

What is deconditioning?

Deconditioning is the effect that disuse has on your body. Often those affected with RA stop using affected body parts due to pain or depression. As a result, muscles become weaker and bones begin to deteriorate. Rehabilitation medicine is directed to prevent you from deconditioning.

What kind of team is involved in my rehabilitation?

Your rehabilitation team will consist of a rehabilitation physician; your rheumatologist, of course; a rehabilitation nurse; an occupational therapist (OT) to help you with your activities of daily living; and a physical therapist (PT). A social worker, a psychologist, and even a speech therapist can be brought in if needed. All of these people may work with you to help improve your quality of life.

What are some of the pain-relieving modalities that might be used?

Both heat and cold can decrease joint pain. Heat can be given by way of paraffin baths, application of moist hot packs, or even immersion in warm water. Cold therapy can be given via ice packs or immersion in cold water. This helps reduce swelling, raise the pain threshold, and decrease muscle spasm.

Topical creams and liniments can be applied to relieve pain. One example is a cream containing capsaicin (an extract of paprika), which is very helpful in relieving the pain of RA.

Electrical nerve stimulation is another method used to relieve pain. This method, called transcutaneous electrical nerve stimulation (TENS), is good for bone pain and even nerve pain in certain sites. Electrodes that transmit mild electrical impulses are attached to the skin. These electrical impulses are thought to relieve pain by interrupting the pain pathway, by increasing the production of endorphins, or by increasing the blood supply to the affected area. Though this procedure is relatively painless, a mild tingling or massaging sensation is felt as the electrical impulses are emitted.

Are there specific treatments for different parts of the body?

Absolutely. Rehabilitation therapy can strengthen each area with specific exercises and assist devices. One such device to aid function is the splint. There are resting splints, which basically immobilize a part of the body like the hand or the wrist, and functional splints, which are designed to support a limb during activities, such as the hands during exercises or the knees while walking.

8

◆

Alternative Therapies

In addition to the several traditional methods of treating the symptoms of rheumatoid arthritis, there are quite a few alternative therapies that many people use. If you choose to try alternative therapies, do not abandon traditional medicine altogether; instead, talk to your doctor about integrating these therapies into your health-care regimen. This is called complementary medicine. Never use any therapy without first discussing it with your doctor. It might adversely interact with any medicines you are already taking.

What is alternative medicine?

Those therapies outside the realm of traditional medicine are considered alternative medicine. These include herbal medicines, homeopathy, mind-body medicines, traditional Chinese medicine, and many others.

What can complementary medicine do for me?

Combining alternative and traditional therapies, if nothing else, helps get you involved in your own health care, as you research different therapies and providers. In addition, there are many who find relief through adding alternative therapies to their traditional health care.

Should I tell my doctor that I am undergoing any alternative treatment?

Yes, you should tell your doctor in detail about any treatment undergone outside of his or her care. Even if you are concerned that your doctor will not approve, it is very important to let him or her know about anything that you are taking—even vitamins or other nutritional supplements or antacids. Almost anything can interact adversely with any medications you are taking, so your doctor must be on top of what you take in order to prevent any adverse reactions.

Might stress-reduction techniques be useful in treating my RA symptoms?

Stress certainly contributes to pain; consequently, reducing stress and improving relaxation can, of course, help reduce pain. There are many methods to aid in understanding, coping with, and reducing stress. Some of these techniques include guided imagery, visualization, hypnosis, yoga, qi gong, and tai chi. Read up on some of these relaxation and stress-reduction techniques to see if any of them sound right for you.

Is meditation useful?

Meditation is another relaxation technique. There is much data available that show that meditation and prayer play major roles in both the treatment and prevention of disease. While these techniques may not be for everyone, they have proven to be quite effective in those patients receptive to their benefits.

Is massage good for me if I have RA?

Massage, or bodywork, can be useful in relaxing the muscles and easing tension. By all means, try some type of massage. There are many kinds of massage, so you'll have to do some research first. Whichever type you choose, make sure the therapist is well experienced in bodywork.

Never have any type of bodywork performed on inflamed joints, if you are having a flare of your disease, or where the skin is broken. Massage should not be painful; it should be a comfortable experience.

Would acupuncture be helpful in treating my RA?

There is good documentation today that this area of medicine not only has benefit for you but is also being prescribed more and more by medical doctors. Acupuncture can relieve pain and discomfort for many arthritis sufferers—including those with rheumatoid arthritis. In fact, in many parts of the world, acupuncture is the only treatment available for RA. In many foreign studies, acupuncture has been found to decrease the number of nonsteroidal medications that you have to take to remain pain free.

Should I abandon my medical doctor for acupuncture if it helps me?

No! Never give up on traditional medicine. These medicines have been proven to help you beyond a doubt. Moreover, you may worsen again once you completely discontinue traditional medicines.

Will bee venom help my rheumatoid arthritis?

There are anti-inflammatory agents present in bee venom in addition to those that cause pain. As such, some patients use bee venom to treat inflammation and find it to be helpful; however, there are no clinical trials that have shown bee venom to have any use in RA.

My cousin wears a copper bracelet to help his arthritis. Is it good for RA?

The use of a copper bracelet cannot hurt your cousin, so if he finds relief in wearing the bracelet, there is no reason he should stop. But there is no documented evidence that it is helpful in relieving the symptoms of RA.

Can low-energy laser light therapy help my RA?

Just as the name suggests, low-energy laser light therapy is the use of a low-energy laser for therapeutic purposes. There is no documented evidence that this therapy helps improve RA symptoms. Besides running the risk of damaging your eyes with the beam, it is extremely expensive.

Is magnet therapy any good for me?

I have seen some impressive results with magnet therapy in people afflicted with rheumatoid arthritis. Unfortunately, again, there is little scientific data available regarding its efficacy. If you find it to be helpful for you, then feel free to use it. Do not wear magnets in airports, near your computer, or near nails.

Would changing my diet help my RA?

Diet plays a major role in immune function, so certainly there are changes one can make in his or her diet that might help lessen the negative effects of the disease. Several studies show that fish oils, evening primrose oil, and borage oil are very good for those with this disease. This is due to the essential fatty acids—omega-3 and omega-6 fatty acids. Other overall dietary changes, such as increasing your intake of fruits and vegetables and whole-grain foods and decreasing your intake of saturated fats, sugar, and refined carbohydrates, are always good changes to make, particularly if you have a chronic illness like RA.

What are some of the supplements that are useful in RA?

SUPPLEMENTS USEFUL IN THE TREATMENT
OF RHEUMATOID ARTHRITIS

SUPPLEMENT	EFFECTS, COMMENTS
Black Currant Oil	• Good source of gamma-linolenic acid (GLA). • May help relieve pain, stiffness, and inflammation.
Borage Oil	• Good source of GLA. • May help relieve pain, stiffness, and inflammation.
Boron	• May help relieve pain, stiffness, and inflammation. • May raise estrogen levels.
Boswellia	• Often used in herbal combinations. • May help relieve pain, stiffness, and inflammation.
Cat's Claw	• South American remedy. • In animal studies, relieved pain and inflammation.
Collagen	• Relieves pain, stiffness, and inflammation.
	(continued)

SUPPLEMENTS USEFUL IN THE TREATMENT
OF RHEUMATOID ARTHRITIS (*continued*)

SUPPLEMENT	EFFECTS, COMMENTS
Curcumin	• Relieves pain, stiffness, and inflammation.
Evening Primrose Oil	• Good source of GLA. • May help relieve pain, stiffness, and inflammation.
Fish Oil	• May help relieve pain, stiffness, inflammation, anxiety, and depression.
Flaxseed	• May help relieve pain, stiffness, and inflammation. • Laxative.
Folic acid	• Helps reduce the side effects of methotrexate.
Ginger	• Relieves pain and inflammation.
Gamma-linolenic Acid	• Relieves pain, stiffness, and inflammation.
Green tea	• In animal studies, relieved inflammation.
Selenium	• May help relieve pain, stiffness, and inflammation.
Stinging Nettle	• May help relieve pain, stiffness, and inflammation. • May enhance the effects of NSAIDs.
Thunder God Vine	• Relieves pain and inflammation. • Not much research data on this herb.
Turmeric	• May help relieve pain, stiffness, and inflammation.

(*continued*)

SUPPLEMENTS USEFUL IN THE TREATMENT
OF RHEUMATOID ARTHRITIS (*continued*)

SUPPLEMENT	EFFECTS, COMMENTS
Zinc sulfate	• May help relieve pain, stiffness, and inflammation. • Helps psoriatic arthritis.

© 1999. Reprinted with permission of the Arthritis Foundation, 1330 W. Peachtree St., Atlanta, GA 30309 (with modifications granted by Judith Horstman). For more information, please call the Arthritis Foundation's Information Line at 1-800-283-7800 or log on to www.arthritis.org.

I've heard a lot about glucosamine and chondroitin sulfate in the treatment of arthritis. Is this useful for my RA?

Glucosamine and chondroitin have been found to be effective agents in the treatment of osteoarthritis. There is much less documented evidence of these supplements' effectiveness in the treatment of rheumatoid arthritis. There are several RA patients who swear by these minerals' effectiveness, however. These supplements are harmless and are indeed useful for patients with some cartilage loss, so if you find relief with these supplements, there is no reason that you should stop taking them.

There are some side effects that you should watch out for when taking glucosamine and chondroitin, including nausea, heavy-metal contamination in some products, and a greater chance of bleeding, as this supplement interferes with blood clotting.

Conclusion

While there is still much we do not know about this mysterious disorder, helpful information is surfacing regularly. New, more effective treatments continue to be developed. In addition, there are many exciting and promising discoveries on the horizon. Hopefully, by the time the next edition of this book is published, many of these valuable findings will add to the book's factual content.

It is important to remember that, although there are many emerging traditional and alternative treatments for RA, you must never start a new treatment or discontinue a prescribed treatment without first discussing it with your doctor. If you have a caring physician, he or she will review all the possibilities of treatment with you.

Meanwhile, living with rheumatoid arthritis is a day-to-day struggle. I wish you the best in your efforts to succeed in this endeavor.

Suggested Readings

Horstman, J. *Arthritis Foundation's Guide to Alternative Therapies.* Arthritis Foundation, Atlanta, 1999.

This is an excellent and responsible guide to the alternate drugs and their value in treating rheumatoid arthritis. It is written for the layperson.

Lahita, R.G., Chiorazzi, N., Reeves, W. Editors. *Textbook of the Autoimmune Diseases.* Lippincott Raven Williams and Wilkens, Philadelphia, 2000.

This book deals with all of the autoimmune diseases of which RA is one. There are chapters here on everything relating to RA, such as fibromyalgia and other diseases like lupus and Sjögren's syndrome.

Panush, R. et al., Editors. *The Yearbook of Rheumatology, Arthritis and Musculoskeletal Disease.* (Published yearly) Mosby Inc., Saint Louis.

This series is published yearly and meant to highlight important papers for the primary physician or the arthritis specialist. The commentary given after each selected paper is a candid one by an expert.

Kelly, W., Harris, E., Ruddy, S., Sledge, C., Editors. *Textbook of Rheumatology,* 6th Edition. W. B. Saunders, Philadelphia, PA. 1999.

This is the standard textbook on arthritic disease. It is primarily a reference work for rheumatologists.

Klipple, J., Dieppe, P. *Rheumatology.* Lippincott Raven Williams and Wilkens, Philadelphia, PA. 2000.

This easy to read book is a very popular textbook for physicians on the rheumatic diseases.

Helpful Organizations for People Who Suffer from Rheumatoid Arthritis

The Arthritis Foundation, National Office, 1330 Peachtree Street, Atlanta, Georgia 30309

Lyme Disease Foundation, 1 Financial Plaza, Hartford, Connecticut 06103

Fibromyalgia Alliance of America, PO Box 21990, Columbus, Ohio 43221-0980

Reflex Sympathetic Dystrophy Syndrome Association, 116 Haddon Avenue, Suite D, Haddonfield, New Jersey 08033

Index